CROCK POT COOKBOOK 2021

INEXPENSIVE AND TASTY RECIPES FOR BEGINNERS

RICHARD DUBOIS

Table of Contents

Paprika Pork

INGREDIENTS

- 3 to 4 pounds country style pork ribs, boneless
- 1/3 cup all-purpose flour
- 4 teaspoons Hungarian paprika
- 1/2 teaspoon salt
- Dash pepper
- 1 to 2 tablespoons vegetable oil
- 1 large onion, halved, sliced
- 1/2 cup chicken broth
- 1/2 cup sour cream

PREPARATION

1. Wash pork and pat dry. Combine flour, paprika, salt, and pepper in a food storage bag. Toss pork in the bag and coat thoroughly.
2. Heat the vegetable oil in a large skillet over medium-high heat. Add the pork and onions; brown for about 5 to 6 minutes, turning pork ribs once to brown both sides. Arrange the browned pork and onions in a 5 to 7 quart slow cooker. Pour chicken broth in the hot pan and scrape up browned bits; pour over the pork.
3. Cover and cook on LOW for 6 to 8 hours. Remove pork and keep warm.
4. Pour juices into a saucepan and place over medium heat. Simmer for 5 to 8 minutes, until reduced by about 1/4 to 1/3. Remove from heat and stir in sour cream; serve the sauce with the pork.
5. Serves 4 to 6.

Pasta Sauce with Sausage & Sun-Dried Tomatoes

INGREDIENTS

- olive oil
- 1 pound mild Italian sausage links
- 1 medium onion, chopped
- 1/4 cup shredded carrot (1 small carrot)
- 1 sweet bell pepper (I use red or yellow)
- 1 medium yellow summer squash or zucchini, seeded and chopped (about 1/2-inch pieces)
- 2 cloves garlic, minced
- 4 to 6 leaves fresh basil, chopped
- 6 sun-dried tomatoes, diced
- 1 small can (6 oz) tomato paste
- 1 can (15 oz) diced tomatoes, undrained

- 1 tablespoon water

PREPARATION

1. Brown sausage on all sides in a little olive oil; add onions and saute until onions are slightly browned. Slice sausage; place in the crockpot with the onion. Add remaining ingredients; cover and cook on low for 6 to 8 hours, or 3 to 4 hours on high (you may need a little more water if you cook it on high). If the sauce is a too thick, add a little more water. I sometimes add an extra tablespoon or 2 of water and a tablespoon of dry Alfredo sauce mix.
2. Serve over spaghetti or other pasta.
3. Serves 4.

Peachy Pork Steak

INGREDIENTS

- 4 thick pork chops, about 1 1/2 inches thick, or pork cutlets or steaks
- 2 tablespoons oil
- 3/4 teaspoon dried leaf basil
- 1/4 teaspoon salt
- 1/8 teaspoon pepper
- 1 can (15 ounces) peach slices in natural juice
- 2 tablespoons vinegar
- 1 tablespoon beef bouillon granules or base
- 4 cups hot cooked rice
- 1/4 cup water
- 2 tablespoons cornstarch

PREPARATION

1. Trim fat from pork. Heat oil in skillet over medium heat; brown pork on both sides. Sprinkle with basil, salt and pepper.
2. Drain peaches, reserving syrup. Arrange sliced peaches in crockpot. Place meat on peaches. Combine reserved peach juice, vinegar, and beef bouillon or base; pour over pork. Cover and cook on LOW heat for 8 hours. Arrange steaks and peaches over hot cooked rice on serving platter; keep warm.
3. Strain cooking liquids and transfer to saucepan. Skim excess fat from cooking liquid. In a small bowl or cup, blend cold water slowly into cornstarch; stir into the hot liquid. Cook over low heat and stir till thickened and bubbly. Serve the thickened liquids with the pork.
4. Makes 4 servings.

Pineapple Pork Loin

INGREDIENTS

- 1 boneless pork loin roast, about 2 to 3 lbs.
- 1/2 cup flour seasoned with 1/2 teaspoon salt and 1/4 teaspoon pepper
- 3 tablespoons margarine
- 2 medium onions, halved and sliced
- 1 can crushed pineapple (20 oz), undrained
- 1 tablespoon vinegar
- 1 tablespoon soy sauce
- 1 to 2 teaspoons sugar (optional)
- 1 cup chopped green and/or red bell peppers
- 1/2 tsp cinnamon
- 1/2 tsp allspice
- 1/2 tsp ground ginger

- 1 tsp garlic powder

PREPARATION

1. Slice pork loin in slices about 3/4-inch thick. Dredge in the seasoned flour. Heat margarine in a large non-stick skillet over medium heat. Add pork slices and excess flour; brown both sides. Transfer browned pork to the slow cooker/Crock Pot (3 1/2-qt. or larger). Add onions and peppers to the skillet, stirring, until slightly browned and tender. Add remaining ingredients and bring to a boil; pour over pork.
2. Cover and cook on low 8 to 10 hours. Serve over hot rice. Serves 6 to 8.

Pineapple Pork Roast Dinner

INGREDIENTS

- 1 boneless pork roast (about 3 lbs)
- salt and freshly ground black pepper, to taste
- 1 can crushed pineapple (8 oz)
- 2 tablespoons brown sugar
- 2 tablespoons soy sauce
- 1/2 clove garlic, minced
- 1/4 teaspoon dried basil
- 2 tablespoons all-purpose flour
- 1/4 cup cold water

PREPARATION

1. Cut trimmed roast in half, if necessary, and place in Crock Pot. Sprinkle with salt and pepper.
2. Combine all ingredients except flour and water; pour over roast.
3. Cover and cook on low for 8 to 10 hours. Remove roast. Drain pineapple and reserve cooking liquid. Return meat and pineapple to cooker. Add water to liquid to make 1 3/4 cups. Pour into saucepan. Blend flour and cold water together to form a smooth paste.
4. Stir into hot reserved liquid. Cook and stir until thickened. Pour over roast; serve with rice, if desired.

Pineapple - Cranberry Pork Loin

INGREDIENTS

- 1 boneless pork loin roast, about 4 pounds
- Salt & pepper
- garlic powder
- 1 (1 lb.) can crushed pineapple
- 1/4 tsp. nutmeg
- 1 can whole cranberry sauce
- 1/4 tsp. cloves, optional

PREPARATION

1. Season roast with salt, pepper, and garlic powder; place in slow cooker. Mix remaining ingredients and pour over pork. Cover and cook for 8 to 10 hours on low. Pork should be about 160° on a meat thermometer. To serve, slice and spoon sauce over each portion.
2. Serves 6 to 8.

Pineapple Marinated Pork Chops

INGREDIENTS

- 6 pork chops
- 1 can (20 ounces) pineapple chunks with juice
- 1/4 cup brown sugar
- 2 teaspoons soy sauce

PREPARATION

1. Put pork chops in a plastic storage bag; mix remaining ingredients; pour over pork chops in bag. Seal bag and refrigerate overnight. Put in Crock Pot on low for 6 to 8 hours, or until done. These pork chops are also great on the grill.
2. Serves 6.

Pizza Potatoes In Crockpot

INGREDIENTS

- 3 tablespoons butter
- 1/4 cup all-purpose flour
- 1 tsp. salt
- 1/8 tsp. pepper
- 1 1/2 cups milk
- 1 to 1 1/2 cups shredded cheese
- 5 medium potatoes, thinly sliced

PREPARATION

1. Turn potatoes into a buttered slow cooker. Combine butter, flour, salt and pepper together in saucepan over medium low heat. Whisk in milk gradually until no lumps remain. Heat and stir until bubbly and thickened. Stir in cheese to melt. Put sliced potatoes in crockpot; pour cheese sauce over. Cover and cook on low 5 to 7 hours.
2. Serves 4.

Plantation Pork Chops

INGREDIENTS

- 4 pork chops, loin (1 to 1 1/2-inch thick)
- 1 tablespoon pecans, finely chopped
- 1 1/2 to 2 cups cornbread stuffing, prepared
- salt
- pepper
- 2 tablespoons melted butter
- 1/4 cup light corn syrup
- 1/3 cup orange juice
- 1/2 teaspoon orange peel, grated

PREPARATION

1. With a sharp knife, cut a pocket inside of each chop forming a pocket for stuffing. Combine prepared stuffing with butter, 1/4 teaspoon of salt, orange juice, and pecans. Fill pockets with stuffing.
2. Sprinkle pork chops with salt and pepper; arrange in slow cooker. Brush with mixture of corn syrup and orange peel. Refrigerate remaining corn syrup mixture. Cover and cook on low for 6 to 8 hours.
3. Turn control to high, brush chops with corn syrup and orange peel mixture again, and cook another 30 to 45 minutes.
4. Serves 4.

Pork & Rice Delicious

INGREDIENTS

- 1 to 1 1/2 pound pork cutlets, about 1/2-inch thick
- 1 medium onion chopped
- 1 large clove garlic, minced
- 1/2 cup flour
- 1 tablespoon olive oil
- salt and pepper
- 1 1/4 cup rice, converted
- 2 teaspoons dried parsley
- 1 3/4 cup chicken broth
- 1 1/2 cups frozen peas (or a 10 oz package), optional

PREPARATION

1. Toss pork pieces with flour. In a large skillet over medium heat, brown the chops in the oil, sprinkling lightly with salt and pepper. Add chopped onions and minced garlic; continue cooking until onion is wilted. In a slow cooker/Crock Pot, place the rice, sprinkle with parsley, then add the pork and onion mixture. Pour chicken broth into hot skillet and stir to loosen browned bits. Pour over pork and rice in the slow cooker/Crock Pot.
2. Cover and cook on low for 6 to 8 hours. Add frozen green peas (thawed - I run hot water over them) during the last 1/2 hour, if desired.
3. Serves 4 to 6.

Pork & Cashews

INGREDIENTS

- 1 1/2 pounds lean pork - cut into narrow strips
- 1 tablespoon soy sauce
- peanut oil or other vegetable oil
- 5 cloves garlic, chopped
- 1/4 cup brown sugar
- 1 to 1 1/2 cups roasted cashews
- hot cooked rice

PREPARATION

1. Coat strips of meat with soy sauce, let stand 10 minutes. Set Crockpot to HIGH. Add a little oil to a heavy skillet over high heat; stir-fry the pork just to brown. Transfer pork to crockpot. Add garlic. Sprinkle with brown sugar, cover, and cook on HIGH 2-3 hours or LOW for 4 to 7 hours. Add cashews 30 minutes before serving. Serve with hot cooked rice.
2. Serves 6.

Pork Chili

INGREDIENTS

- 2 to 2 1/2 pounds pork loin or lean pork shoulder, cut in 1-inch cubes
- 2 tablespoons vegetable oil
- 1 large can (28 oz) diced tomatoes in juice
- 1 can (16 oz) chili beans, undrained
- 1 can (8 oz) tomato sauce
- 1/2 cup salsa
- 1/2 cup chopped onion
- 1 small bell pepper, chopped
- 1 tablespoon chili powder
- minced jalapeno or other hot chile, to taste (optional)
- 1 clove garlic, minced
- salt and pepper to taste

- 1/4 teaspoon cayenne pepper, or to taste

PREPARATION

1. In a large skillet, brown pork cubes in hot oil over medium heat. Drain. Place pork in crockpot; add remaining ingredients. Cover and cook on low for 8 to 10 hours.
2. Serves 8 to 10.
3. Good with cornbread or crackers.

Pork Chop-Vegetable Supper

INGREDIENTS

- 6 pork loin chops, cut about 1 inch thick
- 2 tablespoons canola or olive oil
- 2 cans (approx. 15 ounces each) cut green beans, drained
- 1 can (12 ounces) whole kernel corn
- 1 Tbsp finely chopped onion
- 1 tsp Worcestershire sauce
- 1 tsp salt
- 1/4 tsp pepper
- 2 Tbsp cornstarch
- 1 can (8 ounces) tomato sauce

PREPARATION

1. Brown pork chops in the canola or olive oil in a skillet.
2. Put green beans, corn, and browned pork chops into the crock pot. Add chopped onion, Worcestershire sauce, salt, and pepper.
3. Mix cornstarch and a small amount of the tomato sauce. Add cornstarch mixture and remaining tomato sauce to cooker; mix to blend ingredients.
4. Cover and cook on Low 6 to 8 hours.
5. Serves 6.

Pork Chops Supreme

INGREDIENTS

- 1 large onion, sliced
- 4 to 6 medium potatoes, peeled and sliced
- 1 can (10 3/4 ounces) condensed cream of mushroom soup
- 4 to 6 pork chops, boneless or bone-in
- salt and pepper to taste

PREPARATION

1. Lightly spray slow cooker with butter or garlic flavored nonstick cooking spray.
2. Put onions and potatoes in bottom of slow cooker.
3. Top with pork chops, salt and pepper, pour soup over chops.
4. Cook on low for 6 to 8 hours, until tender.
5. Serves 4 to 6.

Pork Loin With Stuffing

INGREDIENTS

- 1 box, about 6 ounces, seasoned stuffing mix
- 4 tablespoons butter
- 1/2 cup chopped onion
- 1/2 cup chopped celery
- 1/2 cup diced carrots, optional
- 1 tablespoon chopped fresh parsley or 1 teaspoon dried parsley flakes
- 1 cup chicken broth
- 1/2 teaspoon salt
- 1 cup dried cranberries, optional
- 1 boneless pork loin roast, about 2 to 3 pounds
-

••• Rub for pork •••

- 1 tablespoon brown sugar

- 1 teaspoon Creole seasoning blend
- 1/2 teaspoon salt
- Dash black pepper
- 1/2 teaspoon garlic powder
- 1/2 teaspoon ground sweet paprika

PREPARATION

1. Lightly grease a 5 to 6-quart slow cooker.
2. Put stuffing mix in a large bowl.
3. In a skillet or sauté pan, cook the onion, celery, and carrots in the butter over medium low heat until softened. Combine the onion mixture with the stuffing mix. Add the parsley, chicken broth, 1/2 teaspoon salt, and dried cranberries; mix well.
4. Spoon stuffing mixture into the slow cooker.
5. Combine the rub ingredients and rub over the pork roast. Place pork on the stuffing mixture.
6. Cover and cook on LOW for 7 to 9 hours, or until pork is cooked through.
7.

   Serves 4 to 6.

Pork Marengo

INGREDIENTS

- 2 pounds boneless pork loin or pork steak, cut in 1-inch cubes
- 1 medium onion, chopped
- 2 tablespoons vegetable oil
- 1 can tomatoes, diced (14.5 ounces)
- 1 chicken bouillon cube or granules
- 3/4 teaspoon ground marjoram
- 1 teaspoon salt
- 1/2 teaspoon dried leaf thyme
- 1/4 teaspoon ground black pepper
- 1 can (4 ounces) sliced mushrooms, drained, or use about 8 ounces fresh sauteed mushrooms
- 1/2 cup cold water
- 3 tablespoons flour

PREPARATION

1. Combine pork and onion; brown in a skillet in hot oil. Drain off fat. Transfer pork and onions to crockpot. Combine tomatoes, bouillon, marjoram, salt, thyme, and pepper in the same skillet, stirring and scraping to get any browned bits. Pour over pork and onion in the crockpot. Cover and cook on LOW for 8 to 10 hours. At end of cooking time, turn to HIGH and stir in mushrooms. Blend together cold water and flour until smooth; add to pork mixture in the crockpot.
2. Cook uncovered until gravy thickens. Stir occasionally to keep from sticking. To thicken more quickly, put liquids in a saucepan and add the water and flour mixture, stirring and cooking on the stovetop until thickened. Serve over hot cooked rice.
3. Serves 8.

Pork Tenderloin Creole

INGREDIENTS

- 2 small to medium pork tenderloins, about 1 1/2 to 2 pounds
- 1/2 cup all-purpose flour, for dredging
- 1 tablespoon Creole seasoning
- 1 small onion, coarsely chopped
- 1 small green or red bell pepper (or combination), coarsely chopped
- 1 rib celery, sliced
- 1 package chicken gravy mix
- 1 can (14.5 ounces) diced tomatoes, undrained

PREPARATION

1. Cut tenderloins in half; dredge in a mixture of flour and the Creole seasoning.
2. Place tenderloins in the slow cooker.
3. Scatter onion, pepper, and celery over the pork.
4. Cover and cook on LOW for 7 to 9 hours.
5. The last 30 minutes, add the dry gravy mix and tomatoes. Continue cooking on high for about 30 more minutes.

Pork Tenderloin with Fruited Stuffing

INGREDIENTS

- 1 package (about 1 1/2 pounds) pork tenderloin
- 3 cups packaged stuffing mix (about 10 to 12 ounces)
- 2 tablespoons dried celery flakes, or 1 rib celery, chopped
- 1 tablespoon dried onion flakes, or 1 small onion, chopped
- 1/3 cup finely chopped dried apricots
- 1 apple, peeled, cored, and finely chopped
- 3/4 cup hot water
- 1 can 98% fat free cream of celery soup
- 2 tablespoons melted butter

PREPARATION

1. Slice pork tenderloins about 1 1/2-inch thick; place in 3 1/2-quart or larger Crock Pot.
2. In a mixing bowl, combine remaining ingredients; spoon over pork slices. Cover and cook on low for 7 to 9 hours.
3. Serves 4 to 6.

Pork Tenderloin Paprika

INGREDIENTS

- 1 1/2 to 2 lbs pork tenderloin, visible fat removed, cubed
- 3 to 4 tablespoons all-purpose flour
- 1 tablespoon paprika
- 1/4 teaspoon salt
- 1/4 teaspoon pepper
- 1 medium onion, coarsely chopped
- 1 green bell pepper, coarsely chopped
- 2 large cloves garlic, crushed and chopped
- 1 cup strong chicken broth (or use 2 bouillon cubes or equivalent chicken base in 1 cup hot water)
- 3 tablespoons red wine vinegar or cider vinegar
- 3 tablespoons tomato paste
- 1/2 cup sour cream

- salt and freshly ground black pepper, to taste

PREPARATION

1. In a plastic bag, toss pork cubes with flour, paprika, salt, and pepper.
2. Chop green pepper and garlic and add to a 3 1/2-quart or larger slow cooker.
3. In a separate bowl or 2-cup measuring cup, combine broth, vinegar, and tomato paste; set aside.
4. Heat olive oil in a large skillet over medium-high heat. Add floured pork and chopped onions. Brown quickly; transfer to slow cooker.
5. Pour broth mixture into hot skillet; scrape the bottom to get browned bits then pour the hot mixture over the pork mixture.
6. Stir mixture well.
7. Cover and cook on low for 7 to 9 hours. Add sour cream 15 minutes before serving.
8. Serves 4 to 6.

Pork Tenderloin and Sweet Potatoes

INGREDIENTS

- 1 1/2 pounds pork tenderloin, cut into 3/4-inch thick pieces
- 3 cups raw peeled and sliced sweet potatoes
- 1/2 cup chopped onion
- 1/2 cup chopped green bell pepper
- 1 can (14.5 ounces) diced tomatoes
- 2 tablespoons brown sugar
- 1/2 teaspoon cinnamon
- 1 teaspoon dried parsley flakes, optional
- 1/8 teaspoon black pepper

PREPARATION

1. Spray crockpot with cooking spray or lightly oil. Combine pork, sweet potatoes, onion, and green bell pepper. Combine tomatoes with brown sugar, cinnamon, parsley, and black pepper; pour over pork mixture in the slow cooker. Cover and cook on LOW setting for 8 to 10 hours. Stir to mix before serving.
2. Serves 4 to 6.

Polish Kraut 'N Apples

INGREDIENTS

- 16 ounces sauerkraut, bag or can
- 1 pound kielbasa or smoked sausage
- 3 cooking apples, peeled, cored, and sliced
- 1/2 cup packed brown sugar
- 3/4 teaspoon salt
- 1/8 teaspoon pepper
- 1/2 teaspoon caraway seeds, optional
- 2/3 cup apple juice or apple cider

PREPARATION

1. Rinse sauerkraut; drain and squeeze dry. Place half of the sauerkraut in a slow cooker.
2. Cut sausage into 2-inch lengths. Place in slow cooker. Continue to layer in slow cooker, apples, brown sugar, salt, and pepper. Sprinkle with caraway seeds, if using. Top with remaining sauerkraut. Add apple juice. Do not stir mixture.
3. Cover and cook on high for 3 to 3-1/2 hours or on low for 6 to 7 hours, or until apples are tender.
4. Stir before serving.
5. Serves 4.

Pork with Chinese Vegetables

INGREDIENTS

- 1 to 1 1/2 pounds cubed lean pork
- 1/2 cup chopped onion
- 2 cans (4 ounces each) mushrooms, drained
- 1 green bell pepper, cut in strips
- 1 can water chestnuts, drained
- 1 teaspoon ground ginger
- 1 cup chicken broth
- 1 tablespoon soy sauce
- salt and pepper to taste
- 16 ounces frozen Chinese vegetables, thawed
- 3 tablespoons cornstarch
- 3 tablespoons water

PREPARATION

1. Brown pork and combine in the slow cooker/Crock Pot with the next 8 ingredients. Cover and cook on low for 8 to 10 hours, or on high setting for 4 to 5 hours. About 45 minutes before serving, turn to high and add the vegetables. Combine cornstarch and water and add to the slow cooker/Crock Pot; stir well. Continue cooking until thickened and vegetables are done. Serve over noodles or rice.
2. Serves 4 to 6.

Pork Chops Abracadabra

INGREDIENTS

- pork chops, 4 to 8, about 3/4 to 1-inch thick
- salt and pepper
- 1 10-3/4oz. can cream of mushroom soup
- 1 10-3/4oz. can cream of chicken soup
- 1 10-3/4oz. can chicken and rice soup
- 1 1/2 cups barbecue sauce, your favorite

PREPARATION

1. In a large skillet, brown pork chops and season lightly with salt and pepper. Place pork chops in the slow cooker with all soups and barbecue sauce; cover and cook on low for 7 to 9 hours.

Pork Chop Casserole

INGREDIENTS

- 1/3 cup flour
- 1 teaspoon salt
- 1/2 teaspoon garlic salt
- 1 teaspoon dry mustard
- 4-6 lean pork chops
- 2 tablespoons oil
- 1 can condensed cream of chicken soup or similar condensed soup (cream of celery, cream of mushroom, etc.)

PREPARATION

1. Mix flour, salt, mustard and garlic salt and dredge the chops with the mixture. Heat the oil in a skillet and brown the chops on both sides. Place the chops in the slow cooker and add the soup. Cook on low for 6-8 hours or on high for 3-4 hours. You can add more soup if you want more gravy. Good over rice or noodles.

Pork Chop Romance

INGREDIENTS

- 4 to 6 pork chops, bone-in or boneless
- flour
- salt and pepper
- 1/4 cup (or less) extra virgin olive oil or vegetable oil
- 1 large onion, sliced
- 2 cubes or equivalent chicken boullion granules or base
- 2 cups hot water
- 8 oz. sour cream (fat free is okay)

PREPARATION

1. Season pork chops to taste and dredge in flour. Lightly brown in oil in a skillet or sauté pan and place in slow cooker; top with onion slices.
2. Dissolve or soften bouillon in hot water and pour over chops.
3. Cook on low 7-8 hours.
4. After the pork chops have cooked, stir 2 tablespoons flour into the sour cream; stir into cooking juices. (It is not necessary for this to be totally blended into bouillon, but don't just dump it on top either.)
5. Turn slow cooker to high for 15-30 minutes or until liquid is slightly thickened.
6. Serve with rice, noodles or potatoes as you choose. The sour cream sauce is delicious!
7. Serves 4 to 6.

Pork Chop & Cranberry Stuffing

INGREDIENTS

- 4 to 6 medium potatoes, peeled and sliced thickly
- 4 to 6 boneless pork chops
- 1 package stuffing mix with cranberries (6 oz) (or add about 1/4 cup dried cranberries to herb-seasoned stuffing mix)
- 1 cup hot water
- 1 tablespoon soft butter
- salt and pepper to taste

PREPARATION

1. Place potatoes in a 3 1/2-quart or larger slow cooker/Crock Pot; sprinkle lightly with salt and pepper. Top with pork chops; sprinkle lightly with salt and pepper. Combine stuffing mix with 1 cup hot water and 1 tablespoon softened butter. Spoon over the pork chops. Cover and cook on low for 7 to 9 hours.
2. Serves 4 to 6.

Pork Chops - Crock Pot

INGREDIENTS

- 6 to 8 lean thick pork chops - 1 inch thick, boneless or bone-in
- 1/3 cup flour
- 1 teaspoon dry mustard
- 1/2 teaspoon garlic powder
- 1 teaspoon salt
- 2 tablespoons oil
- 1 can (10 3/4 ounces) condensed Cream of Mushroom soup, undiluted

PREPARATION

1. Trim chops. In a bowl, combine flour, mustard, garlic powder, and salt. Coat pork chops with dry ingredients. Heat oil in a skillet; brown pork chops well on both sides. Put browned chops in slow cooker. Add soup and cook on low 6 to 8 hours or on high 3 to 4 hours.
2. Serves 6 to 8.

Pork Chops (Crock Pot)

INGREDIENTS

- 6 to 8 lean pork chops, about 1 inch thick
- 1/2 cup all-purpose flour
- 2 teaspoons salt
- 1 (10 oz.) can chicken and rice soup or chicken and wild rice soup
- 1 1/2 teaspoons dry mustard
- 1/2 teaspoon garlic powder
- 2 tablespoons vegetable oil

PREPARATION

1. Coat pork chops in mixture of the flour, salt, dry mustard and garlic powder. Brown in hot oil in skillet, turning to brown both sides. Place browned pork chops in crockpot. Add chicken and rice soup. Cover and cook on low for 6 to 8 hours or on high for 3 to 4 hours.
2. Serves 6 to 8.

Pork Chops In Crockpot

INGREDIENTS

- 1/2 cup chopped onions
- 2 tablespoons vegetable oil
- 1 small clove garlic, minced
- 2 teaspoons Worcestershire sauce
- 1/2 teaspoon chili powder
- 1/2 cup water
- 3/4 cup ketchup
- Salt and pepper
- 6 to 8 pork chops, trimmed, boneless or bone-in

PREPARATION

1. Cook onions in oil until lightly brown. Add garlic, Worcestershire sauce, chili powder, water, ketchup, and salt and pepper. Cover and simmer the sauce for about 10 minutes. Arrange pork chops in crockpot; pour sauce over pork chops. Cover and cook for 7 to 9 hours on LOW heat. Serve hot.
2. Serves 6 to 8.

Pork Chops with Apples

INGREDIENTS

- 6 pork loin chops, about 1-inch thick, trimmed of visible fat
- 2 tablespoons vegetable oil
- salt
- 6 tart apples, such as Granny Smith, cored and thickly sliced
- 1/4 cup currants or raisins, optional
- 1 tablespoon lemon juice
- 1/4 cup brown sugar

PREPARATION

1. Brown chops in oil over medium heat. Sprinkle with salt. Place pork chops in the slow cooker/Crock Pot; combine remaining ingredients and pour over the pork chops. Cover and cook on low for 7 to 9 hours, or on high 3 to 4 hours.
2. Serves 6.

Pork Chops & Potatoes

INGREDIENTS

- 6 pork loin chops, boneless, about 1-inch thickness
- 2 tablespoons vegetable oil
- 1 can (10 3/4 ounces) condensed cream of mushroom soup
- 1/4 cup water or chicken broth
- 1/4 cup Bold 'n Spicy mustard or Dijon mustard
- 1/2 teaspoon dried leaf thyme, crumbled
- 1/4 teaspoon garlic powder
- 1/4 teaspoon black pepper
- 5 to 6 medium sized potatoes, sliced about 1/4-inch thick
- 1 large onion, sliced

PREPARATION

1. In a skillet, heat oil over medium heat; brown pork chops on both sides. Drain off excess fat. In a 3 1/2-quart or larger slow cooker, combine cream of mushroom soup, chicken broth, mustard, thyme, garlic and pepper. Add potatoes and onion, gently stirring to coat with the sauce. Place browned pork chops on top of potato mixture. Cover and cook on LOW for 8 to 10 hours or on high for 4 to 5 hours.

Pork Loin With Cranberry Orange Relish

INGREDIENTS

- 1 large onion, halved and sliced
- 1 boneless pork loin, trimmed of excess fat
- Salt and pepper
- Juice of 1 orange, about 4 to 5 tablespoons of juice
- 1 jar (approx. 10 ounces) cranberry relish, about 1 cup

PREPARATION

1. Put sliced onion in the bottom of the crockery insert. Put pork loin on the onion slices and sprinkle with salt and pepper. If the pork loin is large, cut it into 2 or 3 pieces. Poke the pork loin all over with a sharp fork or skewer. Drizzle with the orange juice then spread the cranberry relish over the pork.
2. Cover and cook on LOW for 8 to 10 hours, or on HIGH for 4 to 5 hours.
3. Serves 6.

Pork Loin With Squash and Sweet Potatoes

INGREDIENTS

- 1 fresh pork loin roast
- 3 carrots, peeled and sliced
- 3 yellow squash, sliced
- 3 sweet potatoes, peeled and sliced
- 2 cups orange juice

PREPARATION

1. Put the pork in the crockpot, arrannge vegetables around the roast, and pour orange juice over all.
2. Cook on low for 7 to 9 hours, until pork is done.

Pork with Orange-Mustard Sauce

INGREDIENTS

- 6 boneless pork chops, pork cutlets, or lean cubed pork loin, about 2 pounds
- 1/2 to 1 cup sliced green onions, with green
- 1 tablespoon oil
- 1/2 cup orange juice
- 1 1/2 tablespoons soy sauce
- 1 tablespoon dijon mustard
- 1 1/2 teaspoons honey
- 1/2 teaspoon garlic powder
- ground black pepper

PREPARATION

1. In a large skillet, brown chops or pork cutlets in oil on both sides. Place chops in slow cooker and sprinkle with the sliced green onions. Whisk together remaining ingredients and pour over the pork chops or cutlets. Cover and cook on low 7 to 9 hours.
2. Serves 4 to 6.

Pork Roast with Sweet Potatoes

INGREDIENTS

- 1 boneless pork loin roast, about 3 to 4 pounds
- 2 to 3 large sweet potatoes
- 1 green bell peppers
- 1/2 cup apple cider
- 3 tablespoons brown sugar
- 1 teaspoon cinnamon
- salt and pepper to taste

PREPARATION

1. Put pork in the slow cooker. Cut sweet potatoes and green peppers in large pieces and add them. Mix the remaining ingredients and pour over all; cook all day on low or about 4 hours on high. Serve with rice. If desired, use a cornstarch and water mixture to thicken the sauce.
2. Serves 4 to 6.

Ham and Cheese Hash Brown Casserole

INGREDIENTS

- 32 ounces Southern-style frozen hash brown potatoes, thawed
- 1 can (about 10 1/2 ounces) condensed Cheddar cheese soup, undiluted
- 1 can (about 10 1/2 ounces) condensed cream of celery soup, undiluted
- 8 ounces light sour cream
- 1 bunch (about 8) green onions, trimmed and thinly sliced
- 1 jar (2 ounces) diced pimiento, drained
- 8 to 12 ounces cooked ham, diced
- 1 teaspoon Creole or Cajun-style seasoning
- 1/4 teaspoon ground black pepper
- 2 tablespoons melted butter

PREPARATION

1. Combine all ingredients in the slow cooker; stir gently to blend.
2. Cover and cook on LOW for 5 to 6 hours.
3. Serves 8.

Ham in Cider

INGREDIENTS

- 1 fully cooked ham, about 5 pounds, small enough to fit in slow cooker
- 4 cups apple juice or cider, to cover
- 8 to 10 whole cloves
- Glaze
- 2 teaspoons dry mustard
- 1 cup firmly packed brown sugar
- 1 teaspoon ground cloves
- 2 cups golden seedless raisins

PREPARATION

1. Place the ham in slow cooker with apple juice to cover and cloves; cover and cook on LOW for 10 to 12 hours. Before serving, remove ham and set aside. Heat oven to 375°. Make a paste of the mustard, cloves and a scant tablespoon of the hot cider. Remove the outer skin from the ham (if there is one). Smear the ham with the paste. Place in a roasting pan. Pour in 1 cup of hot cider and add the raisins.
2. Bake in the preheated oven for 30 minutes, or until paste has turned to a glaze. The cider will have reduced enough to make a flavourful raisin sauce for the ham.

Ham In Crockpot

INGREDIENTS

- 2 1/2 cups diced ham
- 8 medium potatoes, sliced
- Salt and pepper
- 2 small onions, sliced
- 1 green pepper, sliced
- 1 can (10 1/2 ounces) Cheddar cheese soup

PREPARATION

1. In crockpot, layer ham, potatoes, salt and pepper, sliced onion, and green pepper. In a bowl, combine 1 can cheddar cheese soup, 2 tablespoons water, and squirt of prepared mustard; pour over all. Cook on low 7 to 9 hours, until potatoes are tender.
2. Serves 6.

Ham and Hash Browns

INGREDIENTS

- 1 large package frozen hash brown potatoes (32 ounces)
- 1 can (10 3/4 ounces) condensed cream of mushroom soup
- 2 cups shredded sharp Cheddar cheese
- 1 can (10 3/4) ounces condensed Cheddar cheese soup
- 1 to 2 cups frozen green peas
- 1 cup milk
- 1 can ham, corned beef, or Spam, diced, about 1 to 2 cups
- salt and pepper

PREPARATION

1. Mix all ingredients in a slow cooker and season to taste with salt and pepper. Cover and cook on High 4 hours or Low 8 hours.
2. Serves 6 to 8.

Ham & Noodle Casserole

INGREDIENTS

- 1 cup uncooked noodles
- vegetable oil
- 1 cup cooked cubed ham
- 1 can (10 3/4 ounces) condensed cream of chicken soup
- 1 can (12 to 16 ounces) whole kernel corn, drained
- 1 tablespoon chopped pimiento
- 3/4 cup shredded Cheddar cheese
- 1/4 cup chopped green pepper
- dash ground black pepper, or to taste

PREPARATION

1. Cook noodles in salted boiling water according to package directions until barely tender, about 5 to 6 minutes. Drain and toss the cooked noodles with 2 to 3 teaspoons of vegetable oil, just enough to coat. Add noodles, ham, cream of chicken soup, corn, pimiento, cheese, ground pepper, and green bell pepper to a greased crockpot; stir gently to mix. Cover and cook on LOW setting 6 to 7 hours. Taste and adjust seasonings.
2. Serves 3 to 4.

Ham & Parmesan Potatoes

INGREDIENTS

- 4 to 6 medium potatoes, cut in 1/2-inch cubes (about 6 cups)
- 1 large onion, coarsely chopped
- 1 ham steak (about 3/4 lb), diced
- pepper, to taste
- 1/2 teaspoon dried parsley flakes
- 1/2 teaspoon celery seed
- 3/4 cup fresh Parmesan cheese, shredded
- 1 package (1 1/4 ounce) country gravy mix
- 1/2 cup water
- 1/4 cup evaporated milk

PREPARATION

1. Layer potatoes, onions, and ham, sprinkling seasonings, shredded cheese, and gravy mix on each layer. Add water; cover and cook for about 7 to 9 hours on low or 4 to 5 hours on high. Gently stir in evaporated milk and serve.
2. Serves 4.

Ham & Vegetable Casserole

INGREDIENTS

- 4 to 6 potatoes, sliced about 1/4-inch (about 5 cups sliced)
- 1 to 1 1/2 cups baby carrots
- 3 ribs celery, sliced
- 1/2 cup chopped onion
- 2 teaspoons caraway seed, optional
- salt and pepper to taste
- 1 or 2 fully cooked smoked ham steaks, cut into serving-size portions (about 2 lbs)
- 1 can (10 ounces) 98% fat free cream of celery soup
- 1/2 cup light sour cream

PREPARATION

1. Layer the vegetables, sprinkle with caraway seed and salt and pepper; top with ham. Spoon the soup evenly over the ham. Cover and cook on low 7 to 9 hours. About 20 to 30 minutes before serving, add sour cream and stir lightly; continue cooking on low for 20 to 30 minutes.
2. Serves 6 to 8.

Ham in Peach Sauce

INGREDIENTS

- 2 carrots, thinly sliced
- 2 medium onions, sliced
- 2 celery stalks, diced
- boneless fully cooked ham, 4 to 5 pounds
- 1 cup dry white wine
- 2 cans peach halves in syrup, 16 ounces
- 3 tablespoons cornstarch
- 3 tablespoons lemon juice
- 1 tablespoon butter

PREPARATION

1. Place carrots, onions and celery in crockpot. Place ham on vegetables; pour wine over ham. Cover and cook on low 6 to 7 hours. Drain peaches, reserving syrup. Combine cornstarch and syrup in a saucepan. Cook, stirring constantly, until syrup is thickened and clear. Add peach halves, lemon juice, and butter. Cook until heated through. Remove ham, place on platter. Do not carve until ham is cool. Pour peaches and sauce into liner and mix with vegetables.
2. Serve hot peach sauce over the ham.

Ham Tetrazzini

INGREDIENTS

- 1 can condensed cream of mushroom soup, (10 3/4 oz)
- 1/2 cup evaporated milk, or scalded milk
- 1/2 cup grated Parmesan cheese
- 1 1/2 cups cubed cooked ham
- 1/2 cup stuffed olives, sliced (optional)
- 1 can (4oz) sliced mushrooms, drained, or 4 to 6 ounces fresh sauteed mushrooms
- 1/4 cup dry sherry or white wine
- 1 package spaghetti, (5 oz)
- 2 tablespoons butter, melted
- Parmesan cheese, grated, for garnish
- chopped parsley, for garnish, optional

PREPARATION

1. Combine all ingredients except spaghetti and butter in 3 1/2 to 4-quart slow cooker. Cover and cook on low for 6 to 8 hours. Just before serving, cook spaghetti following package directions; drain and toss with the melted butter. Stir spaghetti into slow cooker. Sprinkle Parmesan cheese and parsley over top before serving.
2. Serves 4.
3. Double ingredients for a 5 to 6-quart crockpot, and cook for the same amount of time.

Happy New Year's Day Pork

INGREDIENTS

- boneless pork loin roast, about 3 pounds
- 1 pound of smoked sausage
- 1 pound of knockwurst
- 1 pound sauerkraut, bag or canned, rinsed and drained
- 1/2 cup of brown sugar
- 1 tablespoon fennel, caraway, or anise seed
- 3 tablespoons prepared mustard

PREPARATION

1. Place pork and sausage in crockpot In a bowl combine remaining ingredients and pour over pork and sausage. Cover and cook on LOW for 8 to 10 hours.
2. Eva's Note:
3. I serve this meal with mashed potatoes, green beans and homemade egg bread. It really turns out tender and delicious. I like to spoon my sauerkraut over my mashed potatoes too.

Hawaiian Pork Roast

INGREDIENTS

- 1 boneless pork shoulder roast (3-4 lbs)
- 4 teaspoons liquid smoke
- 4 teaspoons soy sauce
- 2 ripe bananas, unpeeled
- 1/2 cup water

PREPARATION

1. Place the pork roast on a 22" x 18" piece of heavy-duty aluminum foil. Combine liquid smoke and the soy sauce; sprinkle over the roast. Wash the unpeeled bananas and place one on each side of the pork roast. Pull sides of foil up around pork roast; add water and seal foil tightly; wrap again with another large piece of foil. Place in a shallow baking pan or bowl; refrigerate overnight, turning several times.
2. Place the foil-wrapped meat in crockpot; cook on low for 8 to 10 hours. Drain and discard bananas and the juices. Shred meat with fork to serve.

Hearty Party Beans With Beef and Sausage

INGREDIENTS

- 2 cans (28 ounces each) pork and beans
- 2 cans pinto beans or red beans, drained and rinsed
- 1 pound lean ground beef, sirloin or round
- 1 pound bulk pork sausage
- 1 medium sweet onion, chopped
- 1 medium red bell pepper, chopped
- 2 cloves garlic, minced
- 1 can (4 ounces) chopped mild green chile
- 2 to 4 tablespoons drained jalapeno rings, chopped, or to taste, optional
- 1/2 teaspoon salt
- 1/2 teaspoon spicy seasoning, such as Cajun or Creole seasoning

- 1 cup barbecue sauce, your favorite

PREPARATION

1. Pour beans into a 5 to 6-quart slow cooker.
2. In a large skillet, sauté the beef and pork sausage, breaking up with a spatula, until no longer pink. Drain well and stir into beans. In the same skillet in a small amount of oil as needed, sauté the onion over medium heat until lightly browned. Add red bell pepper and garlic; sauté, stirring for 1 minute longer. Stir the vegetables into the beans. Add chile, jalapenos, salt, seasoning, and barbecue sauce.
3. Stir to blend. Cover and cook on HIGH for 3 to 4 hours, or LOW for 6 to 8 hours.
4. Serves 6 to 8.

Holly's Easiest Ever Kielbasi

INGREDIENTS

- 3 lbs of kielbasa
- 1 bag of sauerkraut, drained and rinsed
- 1 medium jar applesauce (Do not use flavored style)
- 1 12 oz. can or bottle of beer

PREPARATION

1. Mix together sauerkraut and applesauce; put in the bottom of the crock pot. Cut the kielbasa into serving-size pieces and place on top of the sauerkraut. Pour the beer over all. Cover and cook on low for 7 to 8 hours or on high for 3 1/2 to 4 hours. If you are at home while this dish is cooking, feel free to give it a stir now and then. I serve it on long hard rolls with tossed salad.

Honey Chipotle Ribs

INGREDIENTS

- 2 racks baby back ribs, cut into 2 to 3 rib portions
- Salt and pepper
- 1 1/2 cups ketchup
- 1/3 cup honey
- 1/4 cup chopped onion
- 1 1/2 tablespoons Tabasco Chipotle Sauce, or to taste
- 1 tablespoon Worcestershire sauce
- 2 teaspoons chili powder
- 1 tablespoon prepared mustard
- 2 tablespoons cider vinegar
- 1/2 teaspoon garlic powder
- 1/2 teaspoon salt

- 1/4 teaspoon ground black pepper

PREPARATION

1. Heat oven to 375°.
2. Line a large baking sheet (with sides) with heavy duty foil. Place rib sections, rib sides down, on the baking sheet. Bake for 1 hour.
3. Combine remaining ingredients in a food processor or blender; process until smooth.
4. Transfer ribs to the slow cooker; cover with onions and pour the chipotle barbecue sauce over all. Cook on LOW for 8 to 10 hours, or HIGH for about 4 to 5 hours.
5. Serves 4.

Honey Dijon Pork Tenderloin

INGREDIENTS

- 2 pork tenderloins, about 1 pound each
- salt and pepper
- 1 small clove garlic, minced
- 4 tablespoons grainy Dijon mustard or country-style
- 2 tablespoons honey
- 2 tablespoons brown sugar
- 1 tablespoon cider vinegar or balsamic vinegar
- 1/2 teaspoon dried leaf thyme, crumbled
- 1 tablespoon cornstarch
- 1 tablespoon cold water

PREPARATION

1. Wash and trim the pork and pat dry; sprinkle lightly with salt and pepper. Place pork in the slow cooker. Combine garlic, mustard, honey, brown sugar, vinegar, and thyme; pour over the pork. Turn pork to coat thoroughly. Cover and cook on LOW for 7 to 9 hours, or on HIGH for 3 1/2 to 4 1/2 hours.
2. Remove pork to a plate, cover with foil, and keep warm. Pour the juices into a saucepan and bring to a boil over medium heat.
3. Simmer for 8 to 10 minutes, or until reduced by about one-third. Combine the cornstarch and cold water; whisk into the reduced juices and cook for 1 minute longer. Serve pork sliced with the thickened juices.
4. Serves 6.

Honey Glazed Ham

INGREDIENTS

- 3 to 4 pounds boneless fully cooked ham
- 1 can Sprite or 7-Up (12 ounces)
- 1/4 cup honey
- 1/2 teaspoon dry mustard
- 1/2 teaspoon ground cloves
- 1/4 teaspoon ground cinnamon

PREPARATION

1. Place ham and soda into slow cooker. Cover and cook on LOW 6 to 8 hours, (3 to 4 hours on HIGH). About 30 minutes before serving, combine honey and seasonings and mix with 3 tablespoons drippings from bottom of slow cooker/Crock Pot.
2. Spread glaze over ham and continue cooking. Let ham stand for 15 minutes before slicing.
3. Serves 12 to 16

Honey-Glazed Ribs

INGREDIENTS

- 2 pounds lean back ribs
- 1 can (10 1/2 ounces) condensed beef broth
- 1/2 cup water
- 2 tablespoons maple syrup
- 2 tablespoons honey
- 3 tablespoons soy sauce (low sodium)
- 2 tablespoons barbecue sauce
- 1/2 teaspoon dry mustard

PREPARATION

1. Place pork ribs on a broiler rack and broil for 15 minutes. Drain well. Cut ribs into serving size pieces. Combine remaining ingredients in the slow cooker or crockpot; stir well. Add ribs; cover and cook on low for 8 to 10 hours, or on high for 4 to 5 hours.
2. Serves 4.

Honey Ham and Vegetables

INGREDIENTS

- 3 pound fully cooked ham
- 4 to 6 medium sweet potatoes, unpeeled, halved
- 1 bunch carrots
- 1 cup ginger ale
- .

Glaze:

- 1/2 cup honey
- 1/4 teaspoon ground cinnamon
- 1/4 teaspoon ground cloves
- 1/2 teaspoon dry mustard

PREPARATION

1. Scrub the sweet potatoes and trim. Cut in half. Peel carrots and slice diagonally in 2-inch lengths. Place vegetables on the bottom of the crockpot, place ham on top and pour ginger ale over all. Cover and cook on LOW for about 8 hours, or until vegetables are just tender. Mix about 2 tablespoons of liquid from the pot with the glaze ingredients in a buttered measuring cup and pour over ham. Continue cooking on LOW for 1 or 2 hours, basting frequently.
2. Slice ham in thin slices, serve with vegetables.

Honey Mustard Pork Tenderloin

INGREDIENTS

- 1 medium onion, halved, sliced 1/4-inch thick
- 1 1/2 to 2 pounds pork tenderloin, 2 tenderloins
- 1/4 cup honey Dijon mustard blend
- 2 tablespoons balsamic vinegar
- 1 tablespoon brown sugar
- 1/4 teaspoon dried leaf thyme
- Dash garlic powder, optional
- Salt and pepper

PREPARATION

1. Arrange onion slices in the bottom of a 4 to 6-quart slow cooker. Trim excess fat from pork tenderloins and cut each in half crosswise.
2. In a small bowl, combine the mustard, vinegar, brown sugar, thyme, and garlic powder, if using. Coat the pork tenderloin pieces with the mixture and arrange over the onions. Spoon remaining honey mustard mixture over the pork.
3. Cut the zucchini into thick slices (1/2 to 1 inch thickness) and arrange over the pork.
4. Sprinkle with salt and pepper.
5. Cover and cook on LOW for 6 hours, or on HIGH for 3 hours.
6. Baste with drippings about halfway through cooking, if possible.
7. Serves 4 to 6.

Hot Dog and Bacon Roll-Ups

INGREDIENTS

- 2 pounds hot dogs
- 20 slices bacon
- 2 cups light brown sugar, packed
- 1/2 teaspoon ground mustard
- 1/2 teaspoon garlic powder
- 2 teaspoons chili powder

PREPARATION

1. Cut hot dogs in half crosswise. Cut bacon slices in half crosswise. In a bowl, combine brown sugar, mustard, garlic powder, and chili powder.
2. Wrap each piece of hot dog in a slice of bacon; secure with toothpicks. Arrange a layer of hot dog roll-ups in crockpot. Sprinkle about 1/3 of the brown sugar mixture over the layer. Repeat, making 2 more layers, ending with the brown sugar mixture. Cover and cook on HIGH for 4 hours, stirring gently a few times.
3. Turn to LOW to serve.
4. Makes 40 appetizers.

Hot Ham & Asparagus Sandwiches

INGREDIENTS

- 1/2 pound ham, chopped
- 1 bunch asparagus, trimmed and chopped
- 1 can condensed cream of asparagus soup
- 8 ounces smoked Gouda cheese, cubed
- 4 green onions (scallions with green), sliced
- 1/4 cup chopped sweet red pepper or pimiento

PREPARATION

1. Combine ham and asparagus and all remaining ingredients in the slow cooker/Crock Pot. Cover and cook on LOW for 3 to 4 hours. Serve hot over croissants or toast points.
2. Serves 4.

Hot and Spicy Pork Chops

INGREDIENTS

- 2 ribs celery, sliced
- 1 cup chopped onion
- 6 to 8 boneless pork chops, about 3/4 to 1-inch thick
- 1 green bell pepper, cut in strips
- 1 red bell pepper, cut in strips
- 1/2 teaspoon coarsely ground black pepper or seasoned pepper
- 1/4 teaspoon cayenne pepper, optional
- 2 cups spicy V-8 vegetable juice or V-8 and 1/4 teaspoon cayenne pepper
- 2 tablespoons cornstarch, blended with 2 tablespoons cold water

PREPARATION

1. Place celery and chopped onion in crockpot. Trim excess fat from pork chops; add to slow cooker. Sprinkle pepper strips around and between pork chops. Pour V-8 juice over all. Cover and cook on LOW for 6 hours. With a slotted spoon, transfer pork chops and vegetables to a platter; keep warm.
2. Strain remaining juices into a measuring cup; skim off fat. Measure 2 cups of liquid into a saucepan. Stir in the cornstarch and water mixture.
3. Cook, stirring, over medium heat until thickened and bubbly. Continue cooking for 2 minutes longer, stirring frequently. Serve pork chops with the vegetables and hot spicy sauce.
4. Serves 6 to 8.

Hunter's Cabbage

INGREDIENTS

- 1 head green cabbage (about 1 3/4 lb.)
- 1 large onion
- 1 cup diced uncooked bacon
- 1 cup ground or finely diced beef
- 1 cup ground or finely diced pork
- 1 1/2 teaspoons salt
- 1 1/2 teaspoons ground black pepper
- 3 cups quartered and sliced red potatoes, about 1/4-inch thickness
- 1 cup beef stock

PREPARATION

1. Wash cabbage and shred. Peel the onion and slice finely. In a large frying pan or Dutch oven, fry the bacon to render. Add the onions and sauté until wilted. Add beef, pork, salt and pepper, and continue to cook until meat is no longer pink. Add cabbage, potatoes and beef stock. Cover and cook over low heat until the potatoes are fork tender; approximately 30 minutes.
2. Serves 4 to 6.

Goulash

INGREDIENTS

- 2 bacon slices, diced
- 1 cup chopped onion
- 1 1/2 to 2 pounds lean pork, cut in 1-inch cubes (or a mixture of pork and beef)
- 2 tablespoons sweet Hungarian paprika
- 1/2 teaspoon caraway seeds
- 1/2 cup dry white wine
- 4 medium red potatoes, cut in 1-inch cubes
- 1 large green bell pepper, cut in 1-inch pieces
- 1/2 cup chicken broth
- 1 1/2 cups sauerkraut, rinsed and squeezed dry
- 1 large tomato, diced
- 8 ounces light sour cream

- salt and pepper to taste

PREPARATION

1. In a large skillet, cook bacon and onion over medium heat, stirring, until bacon is crisp.
2. Place pork (and beef, if used) in Crock Pot with the paprika, caraway seeds, wine, potatoes, peppers, broth, and sauerkraut. Add bacon and onions and mix well.
3. Cover and cook on low from 8 to 10 hours.
4. About 15 to 20 minutes before done, add diced tomato and sour cream. Serve hot.
5. Makes about 6 servings.

Indonesian Pork

INGREDIENTS

- 1 boneless pork loin roast, about 3 to 4 pounds
- salt and pepper to taste
- 1 cup hot water
- 1/4 cup molasses
- 1/4 cup prepared mustard
- 1/4 cup vinegar
- 1/4 cup orange marmalade
- 1 teaspoon grated orange or lemon peel
- 1/4 teaspoon ground ginger

PREPARATION

1. Place metal rack or trivet in bottom of slow cooker or Crock Pot. Or make a "rack" with a few strips of crumpled foil.
2. Sprinkle the pork roast all over with salt and freshly ground black pepper; place on the rack. Pour hot water around pork roast.
3. Cover and cook on LOW for 5 to 7 hours, or until the pork registers at least 145° F on an instant-read food thermometer inserted in the thickest part of the roast.
4. Transfer the roast to a roasting pan with rack or rack of broiler pan.
5. Heat the oven to 400° F.
6. Combine remaining ingredients in a saucepan and stir to combine. Heat until the mixture begins to simmer.
7. Brush some of the glaze mixture over the roast and put it in the oven. Roast the pork for 30 to 45 minutes, brushing with the sauce frequently.
8. Makes 6 to 8 servings.

Island Pork

INGREDIENTS

- 3 pounds boneless pork roast
- 5 to 6 whole cloves
- 1/2 teaspoon nutmeg
- 1/4 teaspoon paprika
- 1/4 cup ketchup
- 2 tablespoon orange juice
- 2 tablespoons honey
- 1 tablespoon soy sauce
- 2 teaspoon lemon juice
- 1/2 teaspoon kitchen bouquet (gravy enhancer)

PREPARATION

1. Stud meat with cloves. Place roast in slow cooker; sprinkle with paprika and nutmeg. Combine remaining ingredients and pour over roast. Cover and cook on low 9 to 11 hours. (high 4 to 5 hours) Remove roast. If desired, thicken juices with 1 1/2 tablespoons cornstarch and 2 tablespoons water; turn to HIGH and cook until thickened.

Lightning Source UK Ltd.
Milton Keynes UK
UKHW020214080521
383350UK00003B/298

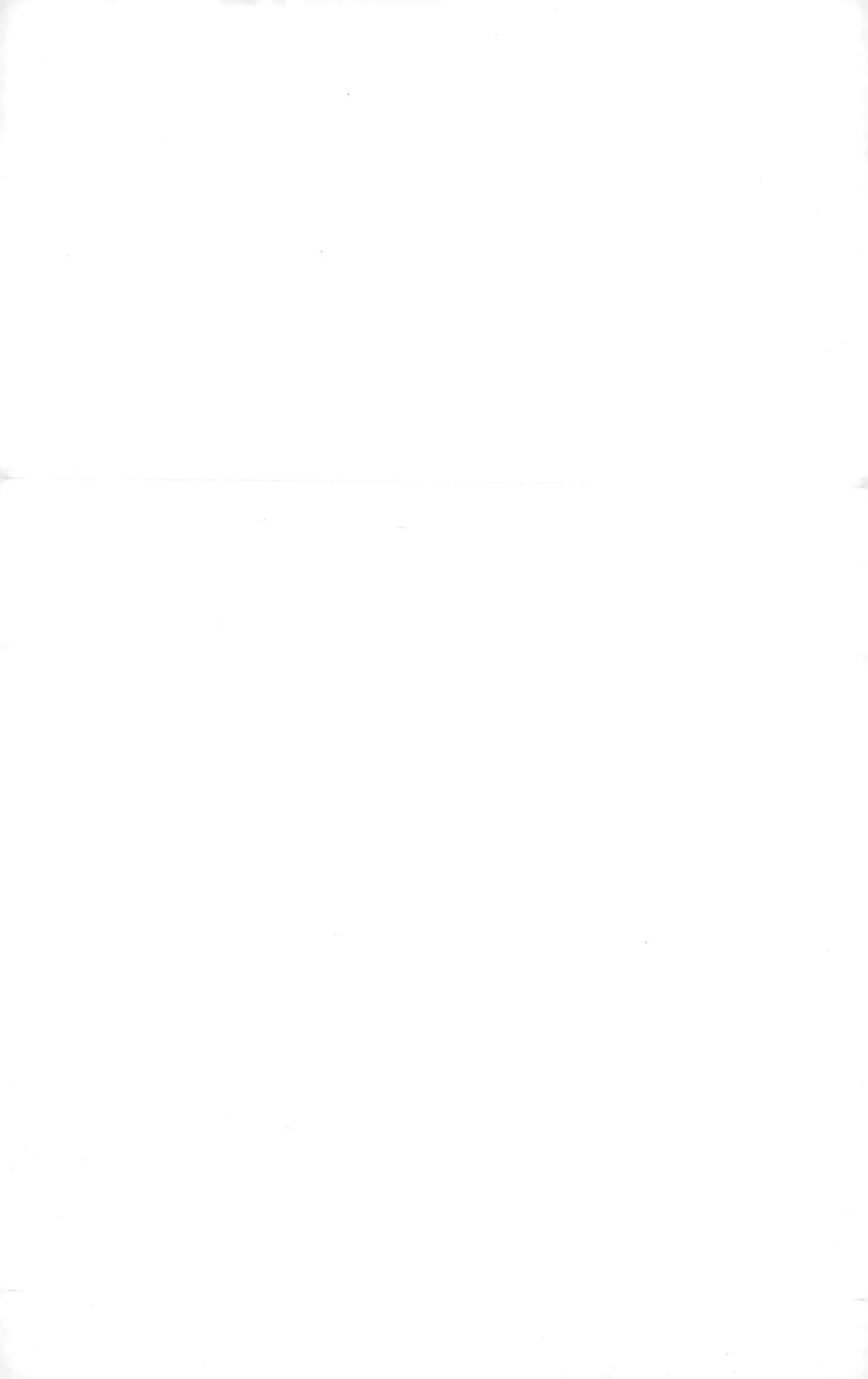